Contents

Introduction

The greatest asset that the NHS possesses is its staff - yet they are also its biggest cost. Of the £124 billion spent by the NHS in England, 65% goes towards employing people.[1]

As the NHS celebrates its 70th anniversary, the question of its funding has assumed centre stage in the political debate, culminating in the recent announcement by the Government of a 3.4% real-terms annual increase over the next five years.[2]

It is critical to ensure that this new money is spent wisely. The Government has asked NHS leaders to put forward a 10-year plan for the health service's future. The Centre for Policy Studies, meanwhile, has called for something more ambitious: the establishment of a cross-party Royal Commission to help make the NHS fit for the challenges of the 21st century.[3] There are certainly huge challenges: how can innovation and excellence be scaled, entrepreneurialism unleashed, new ways of working established and productivity increased - all while maintaining national standards but avoiding excessive central control?

To see the pressing need for such a reform agenda, there is no better place to look than the area of NHS pay - which is responsible, as mentioned above, for by far the largest share of its operational expenditure.

For the NHS to perform at its best, staff need to be properly motivated, incentivised and managed, with salary structures that promote quality care and increased productivity.

NHS staff typically have many differing motivations and clinical allegiances - to their clinical specialty, disease-specific team, site of work, national college, clinical directorate or local employer, all of whom may have different priorities. There are precious few levers that managers can pull to promote better performance, or the delivery of desired objectives.

In other words, to say that this is not a system which anyone would invent is understating the case. The NHS's pay structure is utterly unlike anything seen in the private sector. It entrenches cavernous geographical inequalities, in terms of quality of healthcare staff, between rich and poor parts of the country - or even within individual cities. And the headline figures used in the media to describe NHS pay completely fail to reflect the reality of what people actually earn - with a focus on the 1% pay cap obscuring the fact that average NHS pay has risen by 2.5%-3%, in line with private sector pay.

1   https://www.hee.nhs.uk/sites/default/files/documents/Facing%20the%20Facts%2C%20Shaping%20 the%20 Future%20%E2%80%93%20a%20draft%20health%20and%20care%20workforce%20strategy%20 for%20 England%20to%202027.pdf p6

2   https://www.gov.uk/government/news/prime-minister-sets-out-5-year-nhs-funding-plan

3   https://www.cps.org.uk/files/reports/original/170217121327-AnNHSRoyalCommission.pdf

The NHS currently faces major problems relating to staffing levels. But these - as with many other problems within the health service - are not just due to money, but due to a system that needs fundamental reform in order to make the NHS fairer, more equitable and more productive, both for its patients and those who work within it.

In researching this report, the CPS have submitted multiple Freedom of Information (FoI) requests and analysed a series of NHS databases.

The picture that emerges is of a health service in which the most basic aspects of performance management are neglected; in which pay schemes are inequitable and inflexible; in which there is no way for team leaders and managers to incentivise best practice; and in which bonuses are reserved for senior doctors rather than being shared among staff. Indeed, the NHS may well have the lowest level of use of performance-related pay of any major organisation in the country.

The resulting recommendations include:

- Reform of the NHS's current rigid pay schemes

- Adjusting base pay levels to reflect the relative attractiveness and popularity of particular NHS institutions and the nature of the work

- A new bonus scheme for which every member of staff is eligible

- Objectives that reflect the need for team cooperation to drive through efficiencies and quality patient outcomes

- Organisational objectives set with both yearly and longer delivery timeframes, cutting across individual teams and organisations where necessary

- Better recording and sharing of health data, and better integration of it into the reward system

- The reallocation of current 'bonus' money, plus a component of additional pay awards which would otherwise be applied unconditionally and uniformly

- Discussing overall NHS pay in terms of overall rises, rather than the headline national settlement figure, to avoid giving a distorted picture of salary progression and discouraging recruitment

Given the scale and complexity of the NHS, this report can only provide an overview of its pay structures, and the most significant problems with them. But I hope it will help move the debate beyond the headlines about funding levels and pay settlements and spur an urgent discussion about how we can better reward and incentivise the NHS's staff.

1. The NHS Workforce

The NHS as a whole employs approximately 1.7 million people - making it, famously, the fifth biggest employer on the planet behind the US Department of Defense, the People's Liberation Army, Walmart and McDonald's.[4]

Total	**1,205,246**
Professionally qualified clinical staff	**640,997**
HCHS doctors	116,605
Consultant (including Directors of Public Health)	49,494
Associate Specialist	2,264
Specialty Doctor	7,833
Staff Grade	394
Specialty Registrar	30,837
Core Training	10,297
Foundation Doctor Year 2	6,570
Foundation Doctor Year 1	6,182
Hospital Practitioner / Clinical Assistant	1,747
Other and Local HCHS Doctor Grades	1,320
Nurses & health visitors	319,962
Midwives	26,331
Ambulance staff	21,775
Scientific, therapeutic & technical staff	156,678
Support to clinical staff	**369,499**
Support to doctors, nurses & midwives	286,312
Support to ambulance staff	16,581
Support to ST&T staff	67,052
NHS infrastructure support	**191,619**
Central functions	91,435
Hotel, property & estates	66,187
Senior managers	10,743
Managers	23,398
Other staff or those with unknown classification	**4,871**
GPs	
All Practitioners	**41,693**
Practitioners (excluding Locums)	39,742
Practitioners (excluding Registrars & Locums)	34,715
Practitioners (excluding Registrars, Retainers & Locums)	34,435
GP Providers	22,593
Salaried/Other GPs	11,979
GP Registrars	5,092
GP Retainers	286
GP Locums	2,192

HCHS: 'hospitals and community health services', ie all staff directly employed by NHS England

---

4   https://www.nuffieldtrust.org.uk/resource/the-nhs-workforce-in-numbers

As of March 2018, the NHS in England directly employs roughly 1.2 million people, with a further 175,000 working in GP practices (see table above).[5] Of those direct employees - ie those working in either hospitals or community health centres - some 9.7% are doctors, 26.5% are nurses and healthcare visitors, and 30.7% provide support for clinical staff.

It is often claimed that the NHS has fewer staff than its equivalents. But in fact, as analysis from Deloitte shows, it is pretty much in the middle of the pack in terms of staff numbers - and tends to have more doctors and nurses per hospital bed.

Hospital doctors, nurses and inpatient discharges per head of population[6]

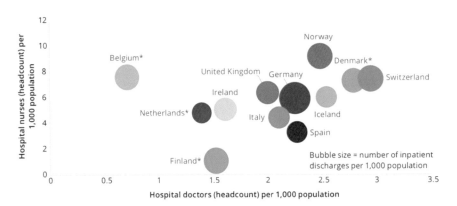

Ratio of hospital doctors and nurses to hospital beds[7]

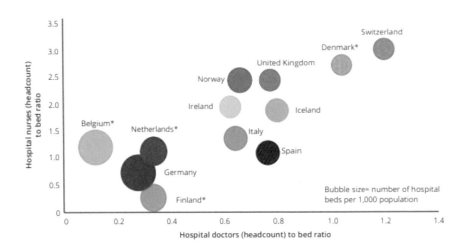

5   https://digital.nhs.uk/data-and-information/publications/statistical/nhs-workforce-statistics/nhs-workforce-statistics---march-2018-provisional-statistics; https://digital.nhs.uk/data-and-information/publications/statistical/general-and-personal-medical-services/final-31-december-2017-and-provisional-31-march-2018-experimental-statistics

6   https://www2.deloitte.com/content/dam/Deloitte/uk/Documents/life-sciences-health-care/deloitte-uk-time-to-care-health-care-workforce.pdf p10

7   https://www2.deloitte.com/content/dam/Deloitte/uk/Documents/life-sciences-health-care/deloitte-uk-time-to-care-health-care-workforce.pdf p10

When it comes to pay, OECD figures show that the UK tends - by international standards - to pay slightly more than its peers to its doctors and slightly less to its nurses.

Remuneration of doctors vs average wage[8]

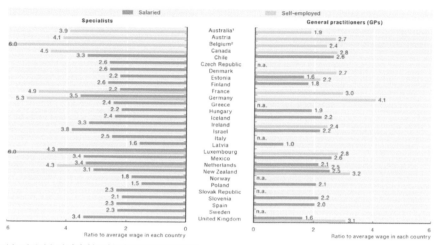

Remuneration of nurses vs average wage[9]

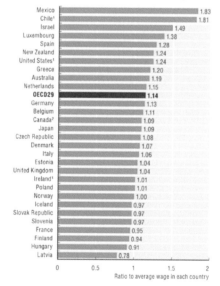
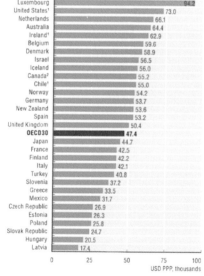

---

8   https://read.oecd-ilibrary.org/social-issues-migration-health/health-at-a-glance-2017__health__glance-2017-en p157

9   https://read.oecd-ilibrary.org/social-issues-migration-health/health-at-a-glance-2017__health__glance-2017-en p163

The Labour Party recently claimed, as a result of FoI requests, that the NHS was short of 42,855 nurses, 11,187 doctors and 12,219 nurse support workers.[10] Retention of nurses and midwives is a particularly urgent challenge, with 29,000 (5% of the total) leaving in 2016-17.[11]

It is, therefore, vitally important that the NHS finds ways to incentivise staff to stay in the profession and not retire early, shift professions or emigrate. The same Deloitte report referenced above noted that:

Doctors and nurses are more likely to move from one country to another than individuals in any other highly regulated profession. Income differentials, as well as wider professional opportunities, are the main drivers of migration.

It added:

There was also growing recognition [in the research for the report] that the global market for talent was shrinking and that looking to international recruitment to fill vacancies was not sustainable in the long term.[12]

The UK, indeed, has traditionally filled gaps in NHS staffing levels by recruiting from abroad - as of 2015, some 26.9% of doctors and 14.4% of nurses were trained overseas, both well above the OECD average.

Proportion of doctors and nurses trained overseas, 2015[13]

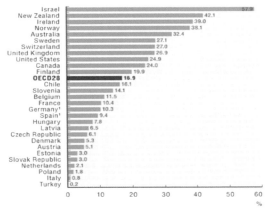

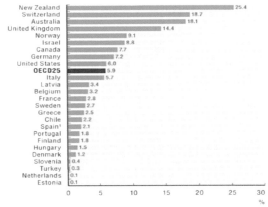

10   http://www.healthbusinessuk.net/news/19122017/nhs-hospitals-unable-fill-vacant-posts

11   https://publications.parliament.uk/pa/cm201719/cmselect/cmhealth/353/353.pdf p12

12   https://www2.deloitte.com/content/dam/Deloitte/uk/Documents/life-sciences-health-care/deloitte-uk-time-to-care-health-care-workforce.pdf p3

13   https://read.oecd-ilibrary.org/social-issues-migration-health/health-at-a-glance-2017_health_glance-2017-en p165

Ministers have recently, and sensibly, announced that they will increase the numbers of overseas workers. Yet we should not see this as a permanent solution, or a way to solve ongoing domestic difficulties.

The NHS has traditionally attempted to predict - in an almost Soviet fashion - exactly how many frontline medical staff it will need, and then train and recruit exactly those numbers, across the various different specialties.

Rigid training structures and accreditation requirements encouraged specialisation, while an ageing population with multi-morbidities is best suited to a workforce with broad and flexible knowledge and license to practise. This command-and-control model also failed to account for staff attrition or any number of other factors.

For example, no one within Whitehall seemed to have realised that as the percentage of female doctors and GPs grew, so would the proportion who wanted to work part-time, for family reasons. (FoI requests by the CPS for this paper show that 88% of male consultants work full-time, compared to 67% of female consultants.)

The resulting staff shortages have led, and will lead, to lower morale and therefore productivity than would otherwise have been the case - not to mention causing more people to leave the NHS, and therefore increasing staff shortages still further.

And while we might take staff from overseas, if we do not ensure we have sufficient staff, and sufficiently well rewarded staff, to cope with the workload, we may lose talent to other countries more quickly than we can bring them in from overseas. Brexit is also likely to have further impacts on staffing levels, or at least on which countries we are able to recruit from.

Nurses and midwives from the EEA joining and leaving the register

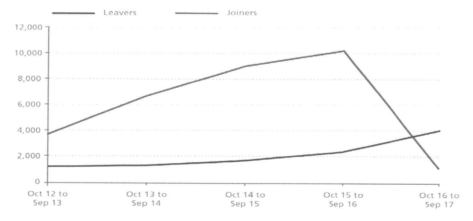

Source: The NMC register, 30 September 2017 (pp. 6-8)

Overall, though, it is hard to argue that the NHS staffing position is hugely different from other countries. Doctors are slightly better paid, and nurses slightly less well paid, and there is more of a reliance on foreign staff. But the key challenge the UK faces is the same as in other countries: to recruit and retain good staff - and motivate and incentivise them to increase productivity across the workforce.

2. The NHS Pay Structure

One of the most peculiar things about the NHS's pay structure - which is very peculiar indeed - is that its origins lie not in Whitehall, but in Brussels.

For decades following its inception, the NHS's pay settlements were agreed via an intricate system of collective bargaining. There was an overarching negotiating body, but various councils and subcommittees oversaw each individual profession - so dentists and doctors and nurses would all have separate deals, and separate terms and conditions.

Among the malign consequences of this system was the fact that female-dominated professions tended to get worse deals, and lower pay, than male-dominated ones. A group of speech and language therapists therefore argued, under the 1984 Equal Pay Act, that their work was of equal value to, say, psychologists and pharmacists. In 1993, in the case of Enderby v Frenchay Health Authority and Secretary of State for Health, the European Court of Justice found in their favour.

Following this, the entire NHS had to restructure its pay systems, in order to ensure that every employee's responsibilities could be statistically quantified and compared. The resulting system, introduced in 2004, is called Agenda for Change - and it covers the vast majority of NHS staff, excepting doctors and senior managers.[14] (Doctors' pay structure is, however, very similar. The highest-level NHS staff are covered by the VSM scheme, which stands for 'Very Senior Managers', as outlined in Appendix 2.)

The full details of Agenda for Change are hideously complicated, but essentially each job is graded against a predefined set of standards. First, the job is evaluated according to 16 different aspects/criteria: 'mental effort', 'emotional effort', 'working conditions', 'analytical and judgmental skills'; 'responsibilities for policy and service development implementation'; 'responsibilities for information resources' and so on.

Within each of the 16, there are then various different levels of responsibility. For example, within the domain of 'knowledge, training and experience', Level 1 requires 'Understanding of a small number of routine work procedures', whereas Level 8 (the top tier) requires 'Advanced theoretical and practical knowledge of a range of work procedures and practices'.

Each of these separate skills then has a points score attached - of which 'knowledge, skills and experience' is by far the most important. (Level 1, above, gets 16 points, while Level 8 gets 240.)

---

14   http://www.nhsemployers.org/your-workforce/pay-and-reward/agenda-for-change

Factor	1	2	3	4	5	6	7	8
1 - Communication and relationship skills	5	12	21	32	45	60		
2 - Knowledge, training, and experience	16	36	60	88	120	156	196	240
3 - Analytical skills	6	15	27	42	60			
4 - Planning and organisational skills	6	15	27	42	60			
5 - Physical skills	6	15	27	42	60			
6 - Responsibility - patient / client care	4	9	15	22	30	39	49	60
7 - Responsibility - policy and service	5	12	21	32	45	60		
8 - Responsibility - finance and physical	5	12	21	32	45	60		
9 - Responsibility - staff / HR / leadership	5	12	21	32	45	60		
10 - Responsibility - information resources	4	9	16	24	34	46	60	
11 - Responsibility - research and development	5	12	21	32	45	60		
12 - Freedom to act	5	12	21	32	45	60		
13 - Physical effort	3	7	12	18	25			
14 - Mental effort	3	7	12	18	25			
15 - Emotional effort	5	11	18	25				
16 - Working conditions	3	7	12	18	25			

These are then combined into a numerical score, which will sit within one of 12 job bands - although, for typically arcane reasons, they are titled 1-9, with 8a, 8b, 8c and 8d providing extra gradations. (The tables below provide a summary, but full details are contained in the Appendix.)

The result of this is a system in which any employee within the NHS who operates under Agenda for Change, whatever their role, can be compared to any other. 'Advanced or high speed driving a heavy goods vehicle, ambulance or articulated lorry' is categorised as a Level 3a ability within the 'physical skills' category - but so are 'advanced keyboard use' and 'advanced sensory skills', such as listening to someone's speech for language defects.

Under this system, a ward sister is judged to be equal to a commissioning manager, and their pay will be locked together at Band 7. Most staff nurses are Band 5, specialist nurses Band 6. Each job equates to a specific band, and therefore employing somebody for a particular role ties them to a particular band.

Band	Job Weight
1	0 – 160
2	161 – 215
3	216 – 270
4	271 – 325
5	326 – 395
6	396 – 465
7	466 – 539
8a	540 – 584
8b	585 – 629
8c	630 – 674
8d	675 – 720
9	721 – 765

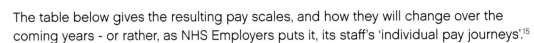

The table below gives the resulting pay scales, and how they will change over the coming years - or rather, as NHS Employers puts it, its staff's 'individual pay journeys'.[15]

Band	Basic Pay 17/18 as at 03.18	Basic Pay 18/19	Basic Pay 19/20	Basic Pay 20/21
Band 1	£15,404	£17,460	£17,652	£18,005
	£15,671	£17,460	£17,652	£18,005
Band 2	£15,404	£17,460	£17,652	£19,337
	£15,671	£17,460	£17,652	£19,337
	£16,104	£17,460	£17,652	£19,337
	£16,536	£17,460	£17,983	£19,337
	£16,968	£17,787	£19,020	£19,337
	£16,524	£18,702	£19,020	£19,337
	£18,157	£18,702	£19,020	£19,337
Band 3	£16,968	£17,787	£18,813	£21,142
	£17,524	£18,429	£18,813	£21,142
	£18,157	£18,608	£19,332	£21,142
	£18,333	£19,122	£19,917	£21,142
	£18,839	£19,700	£20,795	£21,142
	£19,409	£20,448	£20,795	£21,142
	£19,852	£20,448	£20,795	£21,142
Band 4	£19,409	£20,150	£21,089	£24,157
	£19,852	£20,859	£21,819	£24,157
	£20,551	£21,582	£22,482	£24,157
	£21,263	£22,238	£22,707	£24,157
	£21,909	£22,460	£23,761	£24,157
	£22,128	£23,363	£23,761	£24,157
	£22,683	£23,363	£23,761	£24,157
Band 5	£22,128	£23,023	£24,214	£26,970
	£22,683	£23,951	£26,220	£27,416
	£23,597	£24,915	£26,220	£27,416
	£24,547	£25,934	£27,260	£30,615
	£25,551	£26,963	£28,358	£30,615
	£26,565	£28,050	£30,112	£30,615
	£27,635	£29,608	£30,112	£30,615
	£28,746	£29,608	£30,112	£30,615
Band 6	£26,565	£28,050	£30,401	£33,176
	£27,635	£29,177	£32,525	£33,176
	£28,746	£30,070	£32,525	£33,779
	£29,626	£31,121	£32,525	£33,779
	£30,661	£32,171	£33,587	£37,890
	£31,696	£33,222	£34,782	£37,890
	£32,731	£34,403	£37,267	£37,890
	£33,895	£36,644	£37,267	£37,890
	£35,577	£36,644	£37,267	£37,890

Band	Basic Pay 17/18 as at 03.18	Basic Pay 18/19	Basic Pay 19/20	Basic Pay 20/21
	£31,696	£33,222	£37,570	£40,894
	£32,731	£34,403	£37,570	£40,894
Band 7	£33,895	£36,111	£38,765	£41,723
	£35,577	£37,161	£38,765	£41,723
	£36,612	£38,344	£40,092	£44,503
	£37,777	£39,656	£41,486	£44,503
	£39,070	£41,034	£43,772	£44,503
	£40,428	£43,041	£43,772	£44,503
	£41,787	£43,041	£43,772	£44,503
Band 8a	£40,428	£42,414	£44,606	£46,518
	£41,787	£44,121	£46,331	£48,519
	£43,496	£45,827	£48,324	£51,668
	£45,150	£47,798	£50,819	£51,668
	£47,092	£49,969	£50,819	£51,668
	£48,514	£49,969	£50,819	£51,668
Band 8b	£47,092	£49,242	£52,306	£55,450
	£48,514	£51,737	£55,226	£58,383
	£50,972	£54,625	£58,148	£62,001
	£53,818	£57,515	£60,983	£62,001
	£56,665	£59,964	£60,983	£62,001
	£58,217	£59,964	£60,983	£62,001
Band 8c	£56,665	£59,090	£61,777	£64,931
	£58,217	£61,105	£64,670	£69,285
	£60,202	£63,966	£69,007	£73,664
	£63,021	£68,256	£72,597	£73,664
	£67,247	£71,243	£72,597	£73,664
	£69,168	£71,243	£72,597	£73,664
Band 8d	£67,247	£70,206	£73,936	£77,863
	£69,168	£73,132	£77,550	£81,821
	£72,051	£76,707	£81,493	£87,754
	£75,573	£80,606	£86,687	£87,754
	£79,415	£85,333	£86,687	£87,754
	£83,258	£85,333	£86,687	£87,754
Band 9	£79,415	£84,507	£89,537	£94,213
	£83,258	£88,563	£93,835	£98,736
	£87,254	£92,814	£98,339	£104,927
	£91,442	£97,269	£103,860	£104,927
	£95,832	£102,506	£103,860	£104,927
	£100,431	£102,506	£103,860	£104,927

15   http://www.nhsemployers.org/-/media/Employers/Documents/Pay-and-reward/2018-contract-refresh__pay-scales-poster.pdf?la=en&hash=678AD1856E84BE6C6714B7031440AE9EE25638EF

The table below shows the resulting staff distribution:

NHS staff by AfC band[16]

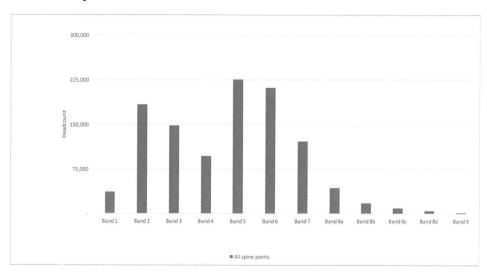

In theory, the advantage of such a system is that it is fair to all staff, and limits anomalies. The same justification is used for paying doctors similarly.

Yet in practice, it is not so simple.

Perhaps the best example is overtime. Doctors, as mentioned above, do not fall under Agenda for Change, but have a very similar pay structure.

The basic salary for a full-time consultant - at least, all those appointed after 2003, when the new contract came in - rises from £76,761 on appointment, depending on length of service. After four years it is £86,369 and maxes out after 19 years at £103,490.[17]

If a doctor chooses to do more sessions, they may receive extra pay, though this would perhaps account for only £10k-£20k, given the limited number of hours in the day. They may also receive significant bonuses, as discussed below. But the real money comes when a hospital is desperate to clear its waiting lists in particular areas, in order to avoid breaching its targets - because it may need to pay whatever it takes.

The table below lists the top 100 highest-paid doctors within the NHS, analysed from October 2016 to September 2017.[18] Note: figures do not include any income from private practice.

---

16   https://digital.nhs.uk/data-and-information/find-data-and-publications/supplementary-information/2018-supplementary-information-files/staff-by-afc-band-and-spine-point-in-all-orgs-on-esr-december-2017

17   http://www.nhsemployers.org/-/media/Employers/Documents/Pay-and-reward/FINAL-Pay-and-Conditions-Circular-MD-12017.pdf p11

18   https://digital.nhs.uk/binaries/content/assets/website-assets/supplementary-information/supplementary-info-2018/ah1864_consultant-earnings-by-age-band-and-gender.xlsx

NHS earnings - the 100 highest paid

	Earnings (£)	Gender		Earnings (£)	Gender		Earnings (£)	Gender		Earnings (£)	Gender
1	739,460	M	26	294,389	M	51	271,909	M	76	261,198	M
2	450,347	M	27	293,016	M	52	271,834	F	77	260,472	M
3	428,737	M	28	292,988	M	53	271,625	M	78	259,493	M
4	400,387	M	29	292,706	M	54	271,550	M	79	259,363	M
5	376,997	M	30	291,351	M	55	270,928	M	80	259,092	M
6	348,386	M	31	291,301	M	56	270,319	F	81	258,765	M
7	337,248	M	32	287,961	M	57	269,656	M	82	258,519	M
8	329,531	M	33	287,743	M	58	269,536	M	83	258,444	M
9	328,821	M	34	285,957	M	59	269,514	F	84	258,254	M
10	327,663	M	35	285,024	M	60	269,000	M	85	258,215	M
11	325,146	M	36	284,208	M	61	268,750	M	86	257,832	M
12	322,559	M	37	281,917	M	62	268,740	F	87	257,449	M
13	322,101	M	38	281,847	M	63	268,523	M	88	257,243	M
14	317,883	M	39	281,616	F	64	268,504	M	89	257,040	M
15	315,236	M	40	278,375	M	65	267,187	M	90	256,685	M
16	312,716	M	41	276,726	M	66	266,864	M	91	255,523	M
17	308,770	M	42	276,716	M	67	266,817	M	92	255,430	M
18	308,708	M	43	276,086	M	68	265,631	M	93	255,356	M
19	307,609	M	44	275,215	M	69	264,560	M	94	254,852	M
20	305,240	M	45	274,954	M	70	264,005	M	95	254,710	M
21	304,934	M	46	274,331	M	71	263,862	M	96	254,280	M
22	301,978	M	47	273,548	M	72	262,962	M	97	254,269	M
23	301,770	M	48	272,925	M	73	262,142	M	98	253,650	M
24	298,116	M	49	272,801	M	74	261,943	M	99	253,529	M
25	295,208	M	50	272,233	M	75	261,738	M	100	253,461	M

These salaries are clearly well beyond the normal salary range. The idea that the extra payments come from waiting list work is supported by the high proportion of radiologists, making up 27 out of the 100, because there is a national shortage and it is a specialty amenable to piecemeal work (as they are paid per scan reported).

But the list raises several questions. Are consultants working at more than one trust, with each employer not being aware of the overall income? And why are nearly all the highest earners male? The first woman is not until position 38 and there are only five in total. It may be that this partly reflects the wider discrepancy between male and female representation at senior level, or between full-time and part-time staff. But as with the differences between specialties, the opacity of the system makes it impossible to tell.

GPs and senior managers

As mentioned above, the payment scheme for doctors is sufficiently similar to Agenda for Change that there is little need to provide a separate overview. When it comes to GP salaries, it is not possible to carry out a detailed analysis as most GP practices are private businesses. The GPs who own the business, the partners, only have to disclose the average salary for the entire practice. Given many GPs work part time, the full-time equivalent pay is opaque.

In general, however, the GP practice receives funding from the CCG based primarily on the number of patients on its list. There is a degree of weighting according to deprivation. The practice is then expected to deliver a core set of services for this money. Further payments are made for providing extra services such as contraception advise, minor operations or care to the homeless. There are also bonus payments for performing certain tasks. These used to be things such as recording blood pressure, but now may be more complicated, such as ensuring a set percentage of a particular type of patient are receiving a particular medication and have been referred to a dietician. The GP partners may pay themselves whatever salary they like after they have paid for sufficient practice staff (nurses, salaried GPs etc) to deliver against this.

In 2005, the average GP partner salary was £110k, reflecting the very generous contract awarded by the Labour government, which also effectively ended GPs working out of hours. Reimbursement charges have gradually eroded this, with a typical salary now being £105k, but some earn £160k and a minority much more.

There is an increasing trend for GPs to take up salaried rather than partner positions and also locum rather than substantive posts. This is because it is less hassle and in the GP-depleted environment they can negotiate higher pay, work part-time and lessen the demands of complex, multiple-morbidity, chronic patients.

Good aspects of the current system include the greater flexibility for CCGs to adapt services through financial incentives, but the self-employed nature of GPs makes coordination and cooperation with other players, including social and hospital care, more difficult.

Although it is not the focus of this paper, there is a strong argument that the structure of primary care payment is no longer fit for purpose: the disruptive nature of online GP services such as Babylon and Push Doctor, which cherry-pick young, digitally connected and healthy patients, will help to force change. Of course, the fact that digital provision of services breaks the geographic link between GPs and patients will be hard to reconcile with the drive towards Accountable Care Organisations, now renamed Integrated Care Systems.

As mentioned above, the most senior NHS bosses are paid under something called the VSM scheme - standing, appropriately, for 'Very Senior Manager'. Base levels of pay for the VSM scheme are given in Appendix 2 - though it is worth noting that the vast majority of NHS managers still fall under Agenda for Change.

The version of the scheme in place before the Health and Social Care Act allowed a salary uplift of up to 30% 'where there are deep-rooted market conditions (or it is impossible to recruit to the post at the basic rate of pay)'. There was also a bonus scheme in which where the top 25% of performers received a 5% bonus.

The current scheme, by contract, is negotiated on an individual Trust basis with NHS Improvement. There has also been a clampdown on bonuses paid, partly to ensure a sense of all staff being in it together, but likely also to avoid negative publicity in a time of wider public sector wage restraint.

3. The NHS Pay Debate

The previous chapter set out the bizarre nature of the NHS pay system.

And it is within this context that the familiar debate about NHS pay should be set. In all the reporting, we are told about an 'NHS pay freeze' or a 'pay settlement of X%'. But in fact, the full picture is much more complicated - and much more generous to NHS staff - than is widely realised.

Within each of the bands described above there are a number of increment points - what is called the pay 'spine'. Every year, anyone working for NHS England will automatically progress to the next pay point along the spine.

In theory, progression is dependent upon annual appraisal. But in practice the increment is almost always awarded, outside of the rare circumstance (in the NHS) of the individual being en route to dismissal.

The national pay increase, recently 1% per annum, comes on top of this. Therefore, for a substantial number, the annual pay rise has two elements: a pay rise based on the 1% general increase and an increase related to their progression up the pay band system.

The graph below shows, for example, the first yearly increment for each of the bands as an individual progresses from the first pay spine to the second. This would be on top of the 1% annual increase. This means, when combined, the net result would be increases of between 2.73% and 5.84% for those at the lowest point of each band.

First-year pay increase (%)[19]

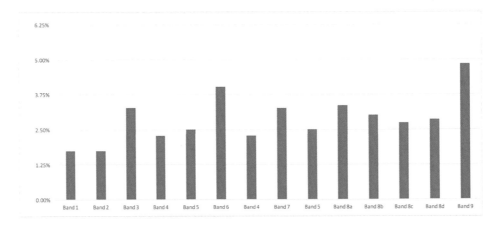

19   This was calculated using 2017 AfC pay band data available at: http://www.nhsemployers.org/-/media/Employers/Documents/Pay-and-reward/AfC-pay-bands-from-1-April-2017---FINAL.pdf, showing the progression of an individual moving from the first pay spine in each band to the second.

The limiting factor here is that NHS staff cannot keep progressing along the spines indefinitely: once the top of a band is reached, a staff member can only get a significant increase in salary by jumping to another band, which requires changing their job description.

However, the spine system still results in very significant average pay increases. According to NHS data analysed by the CPS, in 2016/17 some 54% of staff received an annual pay increment by virtue of progression up the pay spine, in addition to any annual general pay award. (Conversely, 46% had reached the maximum level at any one band.)[20] Alongside its other flaws, it is worth noting that this system discriminates against the lowest paid, with 81% of Band 1 staff at the top of their spine.[21]

NHS staff by AfC Band and top spine point

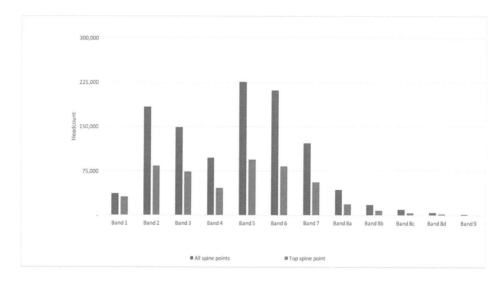

The result of this system has been significant wage inflation. Despite the headline figure of a 1% NHS pay rise, analysis carried out for this paper estimates that the mean wage growth, between 2012 and 2017, for staff operating under Agenda for Change - in other words, all hospital and community heath staff bar doctors and senior managers - was between 2.5% and 3%, with a central estimate of 2.73%. (The full details of this calculation, and the sources used, are provided in Appendix 3.) This compares favourably with mean wage growth in the private sector of 2.14% during that period, and median wage growth of 2.66%.[22]

---

20   http://www.nhsemployers.org/-/media/Employers/Documents/Pay-and-reward/NHSPRB--FINAL-sent-to-PRB-201718.pdf p68

21   http://www.nhsemployers.org/-/media/Employers/Documents/Pay-and-reward/NHSPRB--FINAL-sent-to-PRB-201718.pdf p68

22   Office for National Statics, Annual Weekly Earnings & Annual Survey of Hours and Earnings

Doctors' pay is, as mentioned, technically separate, but also based on pay spines and automatic increments: base pay for consultants, as described above, increases in accordance with length of service from the initial £76,761 up to the maximum of £103,490.[23]

This system has, inevitably, led to efforts to control costs. Over the years, some posts have been downgraded: for example, medical secretaries previously graded at Band 4, with greater associated responsibilities, are often now replaced with those at Bands 2 or 3. But it has also led to efforts to game the system: a popular trick is to write a job description corresponding to a higher band, ensuring that the new recruit will be able to get a change in band, and accompanying pay rise, once they reach the top of their spine.

For both NHS staff and taxpayers, this system is far from ideal. The first problem is that the NHS pay system is inherently inflexible, prioritising length of service over ability to do the job.

The propaganda around recruitment and salaries also damages the NHS as a whole. The current focus on 'pay freezes' risks giving an impression that the pay within the NHS is unattractive - when in fact it is not only comparable to other healthcare systems, as outlined above, but rising significantly more than the headline figure suggests.

The resulting debate can also distort the discussion around how to improve the NHS. If the focus is on underpayment, it means that extra money goes into increasing salaries, rather than capital spending, technological innovation, infrastructure or other areas which have the potential to improve NHS productivity significantly.

---

23   https://www.bma.org.uk/advice/employment/pay/consultants-pay-england

4. NHS Pay: Inefficient and Inflexible

In March 2018, the government announced a 6.5% pay increase over three years for Agenda for Change staff.

It stated that increments would in future be more closely related to performance and appraisal. But much like the much-touted transition to a digital NHS, it's been said before - and we're still waiting.[24]

Yet perhaps the worst problem with Agenda for Change is one we have not yet even touched on, which is its geographical insensitivity and inflexibility.

Unlike most other nationwide organisations, the base pay for all NHS staff of a particular band is broadly the same across the entire country, and all institution types. A physical therapist in Cleethorpes of a given rank will earn the same as a physical therapist in Cheltenham. The same is true, for doctors, of the various specialties.

The extraordinary consequence of this is that a hospital in a deprived part of the country, advertising for a job in an underserved specialty, will be forced to offer exactly the same salary as a hospital in a leafy part of Zone 2 which has applicants beating at the door. To put it another way, there is nothing that poor regions, or poor hospitals, can do to attract the best staff beyond hoping that the most appealing options are over-subscribed.

I am, of course, being slightly unfair. There are, in fact, allowances for regional differences. But these mostly consist of higher pay for those who work in London, to account for the difference in cost of living - ignoring the fact that London is a highly attractive place to seek employment, not least (for doctors) for the potential to become involved in private practice, location of prestigious hospitals and proximity to employment for partners.

Under the current system, employees working in Inner London receive a minimum payment of £4,200 and a maximum payment of £6,469, based on an uplift of 20% of basic salary. In Outer London it is 15% of basic salary, subject to a minimum payment of £3,553 and a maximum payment of £4,528. In the 'Fringe', it is 5% of basic salary, subject to a minimum payment of £971 and a maximum payment of £1,682.

Converse challenges apply to the recruitment of lower-paid NHS staff. Due in part to the expense of living in the capital, or the South-East in general, other areas are, anecdotally, finding it much easier to recruit and train nurses. By contrast, places like Cambridge struggle enormously to recruit because of the expense of living there. This all contributes to inequity of provision for patients across the country.

It can be hard for those who have worked in the private sector to appreciate the extent to which the NHS operates according to this command and control model. In any other walk of life, those institutions or areas that struggled to recruit would be able to raise salaries or offer other inducements. Yet in the NHS, it can't be done.

---

24   For more details on the NHS's digital failings, see the CPS paper 'Powerful Patients, Paperless Sytems' by Alan Mak MP (https://www.cps.org.uk/publications/powerful-patients-paperless-systems/)

The result is that the best doctors and nurses gravitate not just to good areas, but good hospitals. After all, career prospects are far brighter at a teaching hospital with connections to the local university than the run-down district general hospital down the road - and the latter has no way of incentivising you to sign up.

Agenda for Change, in other words, has created several problems. It does not incentivise people to work in less attractive areas or hospitals. It does not incentivise or reward excellence of work: the pay scale focuses only on responsibilities rather than outcomes. There are fewer differential grades compared to the system that preceded it, which allowed more precise differentiation between staff and their levels of seniority. And it is particularly difficult for nurses, clerical staff or others to move upwards: there is a lack of available ranks for promotion and few mechanisms to recognise excellent performance.

Yet these are not the only ways in which the NHS compares poorly to traditional employers. The NHS Job Evaluation Handbook states: 'All staff will have annual development reviews which will result in the production of a personal development plan. Similar to current practice, development reviews will take place between staff and their manager or, where appropriate, their supervisor, a professional adviser or another appropriately trained senior team member.'[25] This should run in parallel with job planning. This too often either

does not happen or is not as effective as it could be. The focus is on how time is occupied, rather than output and does not usually involve an optic from other key team members.

To evaluate the scale of the problem, we submitted a series of FoI requests to NHS Trusts across the country.[26] In most Trusts that responded, the percentage of staff with up-to-date appraisals was between 70% and 90%, but there was significant variation, both between different types of staff within hospitals and between different Trusts. We were told that at Milton Keynes University Hospital, only 32% of nurses and midwives had had an appraisal in the last year.[27] The figure provided by James Paget Hospital in Great Yarmouth was 46%, Oxford University Hospitals 66% and King's College Hospitals 64%.

This is partly because of poor planning, and partly because of lack of incentivisation, but also because of managers constantly fire-fighting and being overstretched with other tasks.

Those managing NHS trusts often complain about the inflexibility of the system. Yet the evidence also suggests that they are not taking advantage of the limited flexibilities that do exist. In theory, high-performing NHS Foundation Trusts do have the right to set their own pay levels and standards, as long as they consult with local or neighbouring employers before final decisions are taken on the use of these freedoms'.[28]

25   http://www.nhsemployers.org/employershandbook/afc_tc_of_service_handbook_fb.pdf p33
26   CPS FOI request results April 2018
27   CPS FOI request results April 2018
28   www.nhsemployers.org/employershandbook/afc_tc_of_service_handbook_fb.pdf p216

The freedoms in question include:

(i) *the ability to offer alternative packages of benefits of equivalent value to the standard benefits set out in this agreement, among which the employee can make a personal choice (e.g. greater leave entitlements but longer hours);*

(ii) *the ability to negotiate local arrangements for compensatory benefits such as expenses and subsistence, which differ from those set out in this handbook;*

(iii) *the ability to award recruitment and retention premia above 30% of basic pay where that is justified, without prior clearance by the NHS Staff Council.*

An additional flexibility is the potential to introduce a bonus scheme in these areas:

Freedoms which must be part of a properly constituted reward scheme for individual, team or organisational performance related to genuinely measurable targets, offering equal opportunities for all staff in the relevant organisation, unit or work area to participate:

(i) *the establishment of new team bonus schemes and other incentive schemes;*

(ii) *the establishment of schemes offering additional non-pay benefits above the minimum specified elsewhere in this agreement;*

(iii) *accelerated development and progression schemes.*

Annex 11 of the NHS pay and conditions service handbook (January 2017) states that these flexibilities are only available to 'three-star NHS organisations'. The problem is that NHS Trusts have not been ranked by a starred system since 2005.

Perhaps it is the intention that such freedoms now apply to 'outstanding' trusts. But of a total of 265 non-specialist trusts ranked by the Care Quality Commission, only five reached that benchmark in 2016.[29]

In researching this paper, the CPS submitted FoI requests to all those hospital trusts which might be or have been eligible to exercise such freedoms. Out of 10 such trusts, only two said that they had used such 'local freedoms', and these only related to the level of expenses and subsistence payments, not overall pay.

To our knowledge, no hospital has ever exercised such freedoms at scale - and if any tried, it seems unlikely that their 'neighbouring employers', ie other hospital trusts, would sign it off. NHS England have confirmed that they have no record of any NHS organisation utilising any of these flexibilities. Moreover, NHS Digital data suggests that none of the 1.2 million staff subject to Agenda for Change have received the relevant bonus.[30] [31]

29 http://www.cqc.org.uk/sites/default/files/20170302b_stateofhospitals_web.pdf p10
30 FOI response from NHSE Jan 2018
31 http://digital.nhs.uk/catalogue/PUB30196
    Staff_earnings_in_NHS_Trusts_and_CCGs___September_2017.xlsx Tab3c

5. The Bonus Boondoggle

The picture that has emerged thus far of the NHS pay system is that it is both highly inflexible, and impervious to local demands or conditions.

Yet there is one element of the NHS pay scheme which at least claims to be responsive to individual merit, or claims thereof - and which, in the process, shows how unjust the current system is.

As for other staff, the pay for hospital doctors is fixed across all geographies and specialties. A doctor's salary in the least attractive specialty in the most undesirable area of the country is identical to that in a specialty and location that are significantly oversubscribed. The pay system, as described above, also involves an automatic yearly increment, as well as a London weighting.

As of March 2018, the NHS in England employed 1.2 million staff. Of those, some 640,997 were clinical staff, and 116,605 were doctors. Of those, some 49,494 were consultants - itself a job title which suggests a certain distance from the interests of the organisation as a whole.

For those consultants, there is indeed a bonus system, called the Clinical Excellence Awards (CEA) system.[32] But it does not operate like a bonus or incentive scheme in the way that most in industry would be familiar with. Instead of being based on the achievement of certain mutually agreed targets, consultants and academic GPs - and only those staff - simply apply if they feel they are worthy. If they don't apply, they will have no possibility of an award. If they do apply, they may receive an extraordinarily high uplift on their salary. And once an award is made, it can very well remain for life.

The table below shows the level of salary uplift that is possible - not just for the year of the award, but for every year it remains in operation.

CEA pay increments

Level	Pay increment (£)	Level	Pay increment (£)
1	3,016	7	24,128
2	6,032	8	30,160
3	9,048	9	36,192
4	12,064	10	47,582
5	15,080	11	59,477
6	18,096	12	77,320

As with everything in the NHS, the CEA operates according to a complex schedule. Levels 1 to 7 are decided by a local committee at hospital level. The CEA committee which decides on pay awards above this largely consists of elected consultants, but with some managerial representation. The levels above this are decided by a national application process. Each of the awards is given by scoring applicants' performance across six separate domains: those who meet their contractual obligations in a particular domain get two points, those who go above and beyond get six, and the truly excellent get 10.[33]

---

32   https://www.gov.uk/government/organisations/advisory-committee-on-clinical-excellence-awards

33   https://assets.publishing.service.gov.uk/government/uploads/system/uploads/attachment_data/file/680513/ Final_Guide_for_Assessors_2018_.pdf

The Advisory Committee on Clinical Excellence Awards only reports on national awards. In 2016 there were 1,200 national applications, constituting 0.25% of consultants. In the last year for which figures for both schemes are available - 2009-10 - the local awards cost £272m and national awards £247m. The BMA, after threatening the Government with litigation, recently secured an agreement with the Government that the number of local awards will increase by 50%, with a budget north of £300 million.[34]

It has, inevitably, been pointed out that the current structure of the CEA is not good value for money and is open to bias towards those with the right connections. In particular, there is no way to link CEA uplifts to the targets set by the hospital where the doctor in question works.

In response, the CEA has now devised a five-year renewal process for national awards. Yet to continue to receive a national award, one needs to score no worse than the lowest ranked successful applicant for new awards at that level in the applicant's region. As the table below shows, reapplication is successful in 80% of cases.[35]

CEA renewal rates, 2016

Total renewal application submitted	416	
Renewal applicants who gained a new award at a higher level	90	21.63 %
Successful renewals	242	58.17 %
Unsuccessful renewals	82	19.71 %
Withdrawn	2	0.48 %

Even better for those receiving them, CEA rewards also count towards the recipient's pension.

In March 2018, an announcement was made on a limited review process post-2021. Those scoring 15 or below across the six domains will drop levels and have their award reviewed in two or three years; those scoring 16-19 will keep their current awards, without review, for at least three years; and those scoring 20 or above will keep them for at least five.

There are, self-evidently, many things wrong with this system. To start with, the awards are recurrent. In theory you could be awarded multiple CEAs in your first year as a consultant and then do the minimum amount of work to fulfil your contract and still receive the bonus for 30 years, plus get a pensionable increase through your entire retirement. And if you changed employer (to a different NHS trust), the new trust would be obliged to continue the previous payments.

Similarly, CEA awards are retrospective and opaque, not prospectively aligned with local needs. Managers have no means of encouraging changes in working practice and incentivising productivity improvements.

Finally, CEA awards are discriminatory. There is no equivalent reward for associate specialist or staff grade doctors, aka 'junior' doctors, or nurses and other staff members operating under Agenda for Change.

The abolition of CEA awards will not, by itself, save the NHS. And it would self-evidently annoy many senior doctors: losses are more painful than gains, especially when concentrated among a minority for the benefit of the majority.

---

34   https://www.bma.org.uk/connecting-doctors/b/the-bma-blog/posts/the-future-of-clinical-excellence-awards-is-now-secure

35   https://assets.publishing.service.gov.uk/government/uploads/system/uploads/attachment_data/file/671213/ACCEA_Annual_Report_2016.pdf p23

But from an objective standpoint, the situation is grossly unfair. No CEA awards are available to 'junior' doctors - perhaps better termed training-grade doctors, given that the typical appointment to consultant level is early to mid-30s. In fact, non-consultant grade doctors make up the majority of NHS doctors.[36] And for non-junior doctors outside the system, there is little prospect of being rewarded: CEA awards were most recently made to 0.4% of associate specialist doctors, 0.6% of staff grade doctors and 0.1% of hospital practitioners, compared to 44.9% of consultants.[37]

Non-Basic Pay for Medical Awards by Staff Group, in NHS Trusts and CCGs in England, April 2017 to March 2018

Staff Group	(%) Staff Group receiving any payment
All staff	1.8
Consultant (including Directors of Public Health)	44.3
Sub-Consultant	0.4
Associate Specialist	0.0
Specialty Doctor	0.6
Staff Grade	0.1
Hospital Practitioner/Clinical Assistant Unknown	0.0
Junior Doctor	
Specialty Registrar	0.0
Core Training	0.0
Foundation Y1	0.0
Foundation Y2	0.0

How does health and social care compare with other areas?

In comparison with other parts of the economy, the NHS uses bonuses far less and also less effectively. Appendix 4 provides a detailed run-down of the various bonus types used in the private sector, which the NHS might adopt as an alternative. But it is clear that health and social care is lagging behind every other industry with regards to bonus structure.

ONS statistics show that the health and social care sector reports the lowest bonuses per employee of any industry, with bonuses per head close to zero.[38] In the wider workforce, a CIPD Survey Report[39] shows that a large percentage of respondents operate group performance schemes as set out below:

1. 47% report profit-sharing bonuses
2. 41% report gain-sharing bonuses
3. 38% report group-based non-monetary recognition awards
4. 35% report goal-sharing bonuses

Productivity in the NHS has traditionally lagged behind that of the wider economy. Indeed, as the Social Market Foundation points out, it is a victim of Baumol's cost disease: 'Despite achieving lower levels of productivity growth, health sector workers expect pay rises in keeping with the wider economy. As such, the costs of delivering the same health service rise over time (all other things being equal).'[40]

Under such circumstances, it seems likely that the NHS could learn from the rest of the economy about how to motivate and reward staff. This needs to be done carefully, but if we are to increase productivity, it is almost certainly necessary.

36 https://digital.nhs.uk/data-and-information/publications/statistical/nhs-workforce-statistics/nhs-workforce-statistics---march-2018-provisional-statistics

37 NHS Staff Earnings Estimates to March 2018 in NHS Trusts and CCGs in England – Provisional Statistics: Tables. Table 3c. Available at: https://digital.nhs.uk/data-and-information/publications/statistical/nhs-staff-earnings-estimates/nhs-staff-earnings-estimates-march-2018-provisional-statistics

38 https://www.ons.gov.uk/employmentandlabourmarket/peopleinwork/earningsandworkinghours/bulletins/averageweeklyearningsbonuspaymentsingreatbritain/2017 p12

39 https://www.cipd.co.uk/Images/reward-management_2017-focus-on-pay_tcm18-34496.pdf p6

40 http://www.smf.co.uk/wp-content/uploads/2018/06/NHS-Innovation-and-Productivity-report-web.pdf p13

6. A Real Agenda for Change

Healthcare delivery is perhaps unique in its complexity.

As mentioned above, NHS staff have many differing motivations and clinical allegiances: It may be to one's clinical specialty, disease-specific team, site of work, national college, clinical directorate or local employer, all of whom may have different priorities.

The goal of the NHS pay structure, like any pay structure, should be to encourage positive outcomes for patients, by encouraging positive behaviours as part of an individual staff member's wider team - for example by focusing on how to increase the number of successful treatments and minimise readmissions.

This is not just about pay, although it is the main focus of this paper. There are also non-pay aspects which are of key importance, such as the lack of proper performance reviews for staff (discussed above) and the tendency of staff to work in silos rather than collaborating across teams and roles.

There are outstanding people who do try to go above and beyond, but hit brick walls because of a lack of broader support. There are many examples of fantastic entrepreneurial and potentially transformative practice.[41] The NHS is not short of transformative ideas, pilot activities and energetic people, but is poor at scaling this excellence and spreading it.

The key in bringing about change is that any reform must avoid introducing a system of pay which is top-heavy, attempts to micro-manage staff, or is too time-consuming. It must also ensure NHS staff can deliver the best possible outcome for patients.

Improving productivity

'Being efficient and thus being able to provide more and better care is a moral duty' - Keith Miles, ex-member, Nurses and Allied Professions Pay Review Body

Current incentive systems in the NHS operate at the organisation level, primarily via the Payment by Results system. This is in fact a misnomer, as the service provider (typically an NHS trust) gets paid regardless of what ultimately happens to the patient. It is a payment for activity, rather than payment for outcomes - which are what actually matter.

This system was introduced by the Labour government in the early 2000s, with a key goal being to get waiting times down by incentivising providers to offer more treatments. In this regard, it was successful. Yet while activity-related payments and targets were helpful in many areas, they had some unintended consequences, including activity-chasing, cherry-picking of easy cases, neglecting other areas of clinical need and fuelling an expensive shift in activity from primary to secondary care which the current government is trying to reverse.

There have been variations on the activity tariff, such as the Best Practice tariff which, for example, might provide extra payment if a patient is seen in a multidisciplinary team.

---

41   See for example https://fabnhsstuff.net

There is indeed good evidence that when better incentives operate at an institutional level, they help drive changes in practice. For example, a recent Health Foundation report quoted one NHS contract manager on the Best Practice tariff:[42]

It really does incentivise people... we go out there and talk to clinicians and say, 'Do you realise, if you do this, we get some extra payment and it really does make a difference?'

We can both monitor productivity more effectively and improve satisfaction for those working in the NHS. For many, job satisfaction involves having variety and appropriate decision-making and support.

One of the difficulties in recruiting to more peripheral areas and district general hospitals is firstly a feeling of isolation from the technical and organisational support available in a teaching hospital (these are likely contributory factors for the reported doctor vacancy rates we have identified of 18% in North Cumbria and 20% in Kings Lynn) and secondly the sometimes more mundane nature of the work.[43]

With the move to Accountable Care Organisations (ACOs) and Primary and Acute Care System (PACS), now rebranded as Integrated Care Systems, where primary, secondary and community care is more integrated, there is much greater opportunity for some flow of staff between specialist units, community and primary care. This would increase both standards and job satisfaction. It is likely that over time, there could be a move toward greater multi-disciplinary teams, both within hospitals and across the NHS more widely.

The exact contours of any new NHS pay settlement would doubtless be a cause of fervent and heated argument. But it is clear from the analysis above that there is a crying need for a system which contains a far greater element of performance-related pay - and that such bonuses should be split between individual, team and a larger functional unit. It is also important that the objectives are achievable and that there is a mechanism for regular feedback to indicate progression towards these goals. Improvements in data capture, sharing and interpretation will be important to facilitate this.

Unachievable objectives are a key source of unhappiness in work and indeed in life more generally. The employee needs to have the resources and ability to meet the objectives and also to have sufficient autonomy to be able to achieve the objectives. Autonomy in how one works towards a goal is an important source of wellbeing and key to retaining staff. The ideal objectives would utilise as many of the employee's skills as possible and align closely with institutional goals.

In place of the CEA, therefore, we should introduce a new bonus scheme that operates yearly, along the lines originally envisaged for the highest performing trusts - but applicable to all areas of the NHS and without constraint.

Every member of staff would be eligible for the bonus. And the level would be based on objectives set at an annual employee review, aligned to core departmental objectives. The goals would reflect the need for team cooperation to drive through efficiencies and quality patient outcomes, based on stretch team goals (eg a team of a consultant, secretary, specialist nurse and their outpatient staff could be charged with seeing X patients over the year, with Y positive outcomes).

42   https://www.health.org.uk/sites/health/files/EffectivePaymentSystemEightPrinciples.pdf p22
43   CPS FOI data April 2018

Any new pay scheme would inevitably need to be consulted on before introduction, but some other possible examples of how a bonus scheme might be negotiated include:

1. A bonus of X% base salary is given to a hospital team (including doctors, nurses, support staff) if patients with condition Y in a catchment area are issued with fewer sick notes AND there are fewer GP referrals. This would motivate the hospital team to educate the community team and improve pathways, focus on self-care and prevention.

2. The local authority has budgeted £Xk for teenage pregnancies for the next three years. If the teen pregnancy team (ie all those who potentially impact on teenage pregnancy) lower the predicted rate by a significant amount, then they would share a percentage of the savings.

3. For other groups, there may be no applicable stretch objective - but a bonus could be structured as a reward for working on a relatively understaffed ward, or for completing Continuing Professional Development in excess of minimum requirements.

It should be stressed that healthcare has a complexity and competing factors unlike other industries, and therefore metrics for a bonus scheme need to take into account these competing factors, focusing on teamwork and quality measures. Such reform should be accompanied by far wider recording and sharing of health outcome data, both within and across organisations, and its integration into the reward system.

The introduction of any new system introduction should be gradual and carefully audited, monitoring for unintended consequences and appropriate adaptation.

However, such changes do need to be made - because they offer the most effective top-down lever to unleash productivity gains in the NHS, improve quality and better reward staff, while leaving the details of change to the grassroots level. Indeed, such an approach could be spread to other public-sector staff.

Greater geographical flexibility

To ensure that healthcare becomes less of a postcode lottery, we need to end the current monolithic approach to salaries, with the exact same pay for everyone, everywhere.

The obvious free-market reform here would be to abolish national pay scales and simply let NHS Trusts pay staff what they like. However, such a change would be highly disruptive, fiercely resisted - and could well result in a significant increase in the total NHS salary bill.

A compromise solution would be to use objective data (such as vacancy rates, patient outcomes, and the number and quality of applicants) to weight salaries according to local circumstances, including geography, hospital and specialty. This might mean, for example, a differential between a district general hospital and a teaching hospital in the same area (since the teaching hospital would generally find it far easier to recruit), or between two similar hospitals in different areas. This would bring market forces to bear on different pay within the system.

I recognise that this would be complex - for example, it is hard to tell whether vacancies in an area reflect bad management, which ensures the hospital has a poor reputation, or genuine shortages of staff due to wider factors beyond the hospital's control (e.g. being located in a less desirable area).

Appraisal and training

To move to a better rewards system, there also needs to be an upgrade of appraisal and training. Job planning should move from the current focus on how time is occupied, to output. There should be much greater involvement of other key team members.

Ensuring greater productivity increases morale

Non-financial factors are also very important for the NHS to address. A recent publication noted:

It is essential that pay rises alone are not seen by Government as the sole solution to the problem of nurse retention, as we have heard in this inquiry that pay is only one element amongst many.[44]

Other key factors were concerns around meeting regulatory requirements for revalidation, workplace flexibility, staffing levels and workload, disillusionment with the quality of care provided to patients and changes in personal circumstances. Feeling valued was a key message, a likely important underlying factor for the junior doctors' strike.

A report by Deloitte also noted:

- *Initiatives that improve recruitment and retention and staff motivation are: more flexibility in career and job planning, including more reliable staff schedules; more opportunities for continuing professional development; and a culture that encourages employee participation, is transparent about decision-making and deploys effective communication strategies.*[45]

- *Where hospitals had been successful in reducing their dependency on agency staff, this has been achieved by building, sustaining and optimising the use of the internal permanent and flexible workforce. Health care leaders in a number of countries mentioned the need to provide employees with a 'sense of belonging', good team fit and clear lines of management to improve motivation and secure the wellbeing of their workforce while ensuring enough flexibility to manage variations in the workload. Some hospitals reported successes in addressing the challenge by introducing new forms of collaboration within and between hospitals in the same geographical area.*[46]

By creating better management which incentivises productivity and better outcomes, we will help to improve the quality of care provided.

---

44   https://publications.parliament.uk/pa/cm201719/cmselect/cmhealth/353/353.pdf p14

45   https://www2.deloitte.com/content/dam/Deloitte/uk/Documents/life-sciences-health-care/deloitte-uk-time-to-care-health-care-workforce.pdf p3

46   https://www2.deloitte.com/content/dam/Deloitte/uk/Documents/life-sciences-health-care/deloitte-uk-time-to-care-health-care-workforce.pdf p37

Conclusion

The NHS's workforce is, as mentioned at the start of this report, its single greatest asset.

If the NHS is to deliver world-class healthcare, and address staffing shortages both present and future, then it needs to enact mechanisms that facilitate grassroots change, and do a better job of recruiting, rewarding and motivating its staff.

As with any system, it can be tempting simply to carry on with what is already in place, while making minor attempts to improve matters. But this report has shown why that must not happen. True, this will be a big problem to grapple with - one perfectly suited to the kind of rigorous, non-partisan consideration that a Royal Commission could offer. But if we ignore the problems with the NHS's pay structures, we will be wasting not just money, but lives.

Ahead of such reforms, there are already important things that can be done. Ministers and NHS leaders should explore ways to make the NHS pay system less geographically inflexible, in order to address the serious recruitment problems that many hospitals and regions face. They should begin the process of reforming the CEA - extending bonuses beyond the consultant class, but tying them far more to performance according to the goals set by senior leadership.

They should ensure that appraisals and performance reviews are taking place as they should. They should consider how Agenda for Change can begin to incentivise and reward excellence - and prioritise outcomes rather than paper qualifications. And they should ensure that public discussion of NHS pay, and the figures published by the Department of Health and Social Care and other public bodies, reflects the reality of how much money staff are actually taking home, rather than the headline figure negotiated with government: the 2.5%-3%, rather than the 1%.

Appendix 1

Agenda for Change grading process

The NHS Job Evaluation Handbook goes through a prescriptive process for grading and assigning scores for the following aspects of work:

1. Communication and relationship skills

2. Knowledge, training and experience

3. Analytical and judgemental skills

4. Planning and organisational skills

5. Physical skills

6. Responsibilities for patient/client care

7. Responsibilities for policy and service development implementation

8. Responsibilities for financial and physical resources

9. Responsibilities for human resources (HR)

10. Responsibilities for information resources

11. Responsibilities for research and development

12. Freedom to act

13. Physical effort

14. Mental effort

15. Emotional effort

16. Working conditions

For example, in the domain of 'Knowledge, training and experience':

Level 1	Understanding of a small number of routine work procedures which could be gained through a short induction period or on the job instruction.
Level 2	Understanding of a range of routine work procedures possibly outside immediate work area, which would require job training and a period of induction.
Level 3	Understanding of a range of work procedures and practices, some of which are non-routine, which require a base level of theoretical knowledge. This is normally acquired through formal training or equivalent experience.
Level 4	Understanding of a range of work procedures and practices, the majority of which are non-routine, which require intermediate level theoretical knowledge. This knowledge is normally acquired through formal training or equivalent experience.
Level 5	Understanding of a range of work procedures and practices, which require expertise within a specialism or discipline, underpinned by theoretical knowledge or relevant practical experience.
Level 6	Specialist knowledge across the range of work procedures and practices, underpinned by theoretical knowledge or relevant practical experience.
Level 7	Highly developed specialist knowledge across the range of work procedures and practices, underpinned by theoretical knowledge and relevant practical experience.
Level 8	(a) Advanced theoretical and practical knowledge of a range of work procedures and practices, or (b) Specialist knowledge over more than one discipline / function acquired over a significant period.

Or for 'Mental effort':

Level 1	General awareness and sensory attention; normal care and attention; an occasional requirement for concentration where the work pattern is predictable with few competing demands for attention.
Level 2	(a) There is a frequent requirement for concentration where the work pattern is predictable with few competing demands for attention, or (b) There is an occasional requirement for concentration where the work pattern is unpredictable.
Level 3	(a) There is a frequent requirement for concentration where the work pattern is unpredictable, or (b) There is an occasional requirement for prolonged concentration.
Level 4	(a) There is a frequent requirement for prolonged concentration, or (b) There is an occasional requirement for intense concentration.
Level 5	There is a frequent requirement for intense concentration.

As an example of how different jobs receive the same ranking, Level 3a for Physical Skills includes:

1. Advanced or high speed driving a heavy goods vehicle, ambulance, minibus or articulated lorry where a Large Goods Vehicle, Passenger Carrying Vehicle or Ambulance Driving Test or equivalent is required.

2. Advanced keyboard use (Level 3a) includes the skills exercised by qualified typists/ word processor operators (RSA 2/3 or equivalent).

3. Advanced sensory skills (Level 3a) includes the skills required for sensory, hand and eye coordination such as those required for audio-typing. It also includes specific developed sensory skills e.g. listening skills for identifying speech or language defects.

4. Restraint of patients/clients (Level 3a) indicates a skill level that requires a formal course of training and regular updating.

A score is then allocated for each domain and weighted:

Factor	1	2	3	4	5	6	7	8
1 - Communication and relationship skills	5	12	21	32	45	60		
2 - Knowledge, training, and experience	16	36	60	88	120	156	196	240
3 - Analytical skills	6	15	27	42	60			
4 - Planning and organisational skills	6	15	27	42	60			
5 - Physical skills	6	15	27	42	60			
6 - Responsibility - patient / client care	4	9	15	22	30	39	49	60
7 - Responsibility - policy and service	5	12	21	32	45	60		
8 - Responsibility - finance and physical	5	12	21	32	45	60		
9 - Responsibility - staff / HR / leadership	5	12	21	32	45	60		
10 - Responsibility - information resources	4	9	16	24	34	46	60	
11 - Responsibility - research and development	5	12	21	32	45	60		
12 - Freedom to act	5	12	21	32	45	60		
13 - Physical effort	3	7	12	18	25			
14 - Mental effort	3	7	12	18	25			
15 - Emotional effort	5	11	18	25				
16 - Working conditions	3	7	12	18	25			

The total scores are then converted to a job band:

Band	Job Weight
1	0 – 160
2	161 – 215
3	216 – 270
4	271 – 325
5	326 – 395
6	396 – 465
7	466 – 539
8a	540 – 584
8b	585 – 629
8c	630 – 674
8d	675 – 720
9	721 – 765

Appendix 2

Senior Manager pay scale

Small acute NHS trusts (£0 to £200m t/o)	Lower quartile (£)	Median (£)	Upper quartile (£)
Chief executives	141,000	167,500	182,500
Deputy CEO	107,500	117,500	132,500
Director of finance	109,000	125,000	137,500
HR / Workforce directors	88,000	98,000	102,500
Medical directors	134,000	170,000	198,500
Nursing directors	95,000	102,500	107,500
Chief operating officer	100,000	112,500	142,500
Corporate affairs / Governance directors	75,000	87,500	92,500
Strategy and planning directors	92,000	110,000	120,000
Director of facilities / Estates	86,000	89,000	105,000

Large acute NHS trusts (£400 to £500m t/o)	Lower quartile (£)	Median (£)	Upper quartile (£)
Chief executives	190,000	197,500	230,000
Deputy CEO	130,000	155,000	180,000
Director of finance	126,000	140,000	155,000
HR / Workforce directors	117,000	128,000	143,000
Medical directors	170,000	182,000	202,000
Nursing directors	115,000	131,000	137,500
Chief operating officer	117,000	136,000	152,000
Corporate affairs / Governance directors	83,000	100,000	112,500
Strategy and planning directors	110,000	122,500	132,500
Director of facilities / Estates	103,000	126,000	135,000

Med. acute NHS trusts (£200 to £400m t/o)	Lower quartile (£)	Median (£)	Upper quartile (£)
Chief executives	160,000	182,500	202,500
Deputy CEO	123,000	142,500	160,000
Director of finance	123,000	135,000	147,500
HR / Workforce directors	100,000	107,500	125,000
Medical directors	169,000	178,000	199,000
Nursing directors	103,000	117,500	127,500
Chief operating officer	110,000	122,500	146,500
Corporate affairs / Governance directors	77,500	97,500	107,500
Strategy and planning directors	100,000	115,000	124,000
Director of facilities / Estates	93,500	95,000	120,000

Very large acute NHS trusts (Over £500m)	Lower quartile (£)	Median (£)	Upper quartile (£)
Chief executives	195,000	225,000	267,500
Deputy CEO	143,500	165,000	200,000
Director of finance	148,500	157,500	190,000
HR / Workforce directors	120,000	130,000	145,000
Medical directors	189,000	215,000	230,000
Nursing directors	130,000	142,500	157,000
Chief operating officer	141,000	190,000	198,000
Corporate affairs / Governance directors	88,000	105,000	117,500
Strategy and planning directors	112,000	137,500	162,000
Director of facilities / Estates	120,000	135,000	145,000

Specialist trusts focusing on one niche medical area, such as Moorfields Eye Hospital, can apply for a 15% premium on wages, which tends to make these areas more attractive.

Appendix 3

Calculating average pay in the NHS 2012 - 2017

Based upon the data available, we estimate that the average annual pay increase (of AfC staff) in the NHS for the period 2012-2017 was in the range of 2.5-3%, with our central estimate at roughly 2.7%. This was calculated based on the following methodology:

1) Data from NHS Digital on the number of staff at each point on the AfC pay progression scale was used to calculate the proportion of staff at each pay point each year from 2012 to 2017.

2) Because data for 2013, 2014, and 2015 is not publicly available, the overall change from 2012 - 2017 was taken and divided by five to calculate the estimated annual change in staff numbers at each pay point. A simplifying assumption that staff numbers changed by the same amount each year at each pay point was made here. Note here also that pay point 1 of bands 1 and 2 was abolished in 2015. Therefore, staff numbers in pay points 1 and 2 were combined for bands 1 & 2 until 2015.

3) Data from the Royal College of Nursing on the AfC pay progression for the years 2012/13 up to 2017/18 was used to calculate the annual percentage increase in pay at each pay point. Note here that because of progression we assume that all staff move up a pay point each year until they reach the top of their band.

So, the pay increase from 2012/13 to 2013/14 for point 2 of band 1, is the percentage increase between pay point 1 of band 1 in 2012/13 and pay point 2 of band 1 in 2013/14. An example may help to clarify what this means: a person who starts 2012/13

at pay point 1 of band 1, earns £14,153. In 2013/14 they move up to pay point 2, and therefore earn £14,653. This means that they got a pay increase of £500 or 3.53%.

4) The pay increase at each pay point was then weighted according to the proportion of staff who were at that pay point that year. For example, in 2013 there were 1.38% of all staff at pay point 10 in band 3 who received a pay increase of 3.79%, so the weighted average annual pay increase for this pay point was 0.052%. These weighted pay increases were then summed to get an annual average pay increase of 2.73%.

Limitations to our estimate:

- Our estimate cannot take account of churn within the NHS workforce, ie people leaving or joining, as it is based solely on aggregate figures for staff within each particular band. This is why we have suggested a range between 2.5% and 3% rather than an exact figure. However, given that the government has access to NHS payroll data it would be eminently possible for it to calculate and publish a more precise annual figure for the mean and/or median pay increase within the NHS.

- Our estimate excludes staff at the lowest point of each band. We did this because we assume that being in the lowest pay point of a band means that they have joined that band during the year. Some of these staff will have been promoted from lower bands and will therefore have received a pay increase, however other staff will be joining the NHS for the first time or rejoining and will not have received a promotion from a lower band. Therefore, we assume they will not have seen a pay increase.

- It is difficult to disentangle these two groups, thus, in order to simplify things, we exclude all staff in the lowest pay point of each band. Because this excludes staff who have moved up a band, this will probably cause our estimate of the annual average pay increase to be an underestimate of the true figure.

- We also encountered a difficulty when calculating the pay increase for the top pay point of each band. Once staff reach the top pay point of a band they remain there until they get a promotion into a higher band. This means that they do not benefit from pay increases due to progression. Other staff will progress into the top pay point of their band every year, who will therefore get a larger pay rise due to progression than staff who are already in the top pay point. It is difficult to disentangle the two groups, especially since some staff will be promoted into a higher band and so will leave the top pay point.

- To solve this, we took the total number of staff in the top pay point of each band and split them into two: as a proxy for the number of staff who were already in the top pay point we took the number of staff in the pay point the previous year. Therefore, the increase in staff from the previous year served as a proxy for staff who progressed into the top pay point this year. However, by doing this we almost certainly underestimated the number of staff who progress into the top pay point each year, which will cause us to underestimate the annual average pay increase.

- Overall therefore, it is likely that our estimate of an average annual pay increase of 2.73% is an underestimate, and that the true figure is closer to 3%.

Data - AfC Headcount by pay point:

2012: AfC headcount by pay point data can be found at http://webarchive. nationalarchives.gov.uk/20180307192547/ http://content.digital.nhs.uk/7572.

2017: AfC headcount by pay point data can be at https://digital.nhs.uk/data-and-information/ find-data-and-publications/supplementary-information/2018-supplementary-information-files/staff-by-afc-band-and-spine-point-in-all-orgs-on-esr-december-2017

Note: this data includes non-AfC staff, which for the purposes of our analysis we excluded.

Data on pay progression by AfC pay points and bands:

2012/13: https://www.rcn.org.uk/professional-development/publications/pub-004239

2013/14: https://www.rcn.org.uk/professional-development/publications/pub-004405

2014/15: https://www.rcn.org.uk/employment-and-pay/nhs-pay-scales-2014-15

2015/16: https://www.rcn.org.uk/employment-and-pay/nhs-pay-scales-2015-16

2016/17: https://www.rcn.org.uk/employment-and-pay/nhs-pay-scales-2016-17

2017/18: https://www.rcn.org.uk/employment-and-pay/nhs-pay-scales-2017-18

Appendix 4

A guide to alternative bonus schemes[47]

Discretionary bonuses are paid at the discretion of the employer. This means the bonus entitlement isn't written into the employees' contracts. The standard of performance required to trigger a bonus and the amount of bonus paid are flexible. For discretionary bonuses to create an incentive, employees must have confidence they will receive a bonus for good performance. A practical problem in the NHS is a lack of managerial time. With the common refrain from politicians and the press to cut managers and focus on the frontline, this would be problematic. But if silos were broken down, clinicians could take on meaningful team management, and be incentivised to do this through bonus payments.

Non-discretionary bonuses are based on defined performance criteria. The bonus entitlement might be written into the employment contract, so employees know how well they need to perform in advance to receive their bonus. The employer may be legally obliged to pay bonuses when criteria are met. Whereas discretionary bonuses typically reward success already achieved, non-discretionary bonuses are often used to incentivise future performance.

Individual bonuses may be best for incentivising employees to reach individual targets. Individual bonus schemes are most popular at private sector service firms (64%

use them) and manufacturing and production companies (55%). In the public and voluntary sectors, fewer than half of organisations use them on average. Employers are more likely to offer bonuses to managers and professionals (53% receive them) than other employees (45%, CIPD 2015).

Team bonus schemes may be used when the workforce is split into teams with defined goals. Team based bonus schemes have proven to be very popular as they help to increase productivity and rapport within a department. Advantages of this are usually that when a team does well the company also benefits. In addition, a team reward system helps to create a good competitive environment within each department. Team bonuses can be used in a variety of industries such as sales, manufacturing, and retail.

Company bonus schemes may be used for rewarding strong annual performance. Company-wide bonuses are usually discretionary, since many factors can affect an organisation's ability to pay. Every employee is rewarded based on the overall performance of the company. A good example of this is the John Lewis Partnership scheme, where every year every John Lewis Partner (staff member) is rewarded with a percentage of their annual salary.

---

47   https://www.brighthr.com/brightbase/topic/pay-and-benefits/bonuses/employee-bonus-schemes

Metrics used to trigger bonuses in other industries include productivity, quality and target measures.

1. **Productivity bonus:** Traditionally this has been used in the manufacturing industry and is otherwise known as piecework, where the number of items produced over a certain period of time determines the bonus paid. However, recently more organisations have taken this approach, for example by monitoring the number of calls taken by a call centre worker.

2. **Quality bonus:** Similar to productivity, a quality bonus can be assessed on the number of defects on products during a period of time. As with productivity, many industries are now taking this approach, for example, by rewarding staff for reducing the number of customer complaints within a supermarket.

3. **Target bonus:** A well-used tactic within internal and external sales environments. Target bonuses are paid if an individual hits a sales figure within a certain period, usually monthly, quarterly or annually. The figure can be a percentage increase on the previous period or a pre-defined target based on expectations.